**My Journey Without Mom
Hugging The Pain,
Releasing The Grief,
Finding Peace and Happiness**

BY MS. CHRISTINE JONES, M.A.

Copyright

John Red Publishing Inc.

Copyright © Christine Jones M. A., 2018

All rights reserved. No part of this book may be reproduced in any form without the written permission from the author at www.thechristinejones.com. Published 2018

ISBN 978-172-889-1156

DISCLAIMER

No part of this publication may be reproduced or transmitted in any form or by any means, mechanical or electronic, including photocopying or recording, or by any information storage and retrieval system, or transmitted by email without permission in writing from the author. Neither the author nor the publisher assumes any responsibility for errors, omissions, or contrary interpretations of the subject matter herein. Any perceived slight of any individual or organization is purely unintentional. Brand and product names are trademarks or registered trademarks of their respective owners.

Dedication

This book is dedicated to my father and mother: Jessie and Gracie Jones, and to all my family members, who I love dearly. I appreciate the love, encouragement, and advice you have given me over the years.

I also give thanks, praise, glory, and honor to God who made this terrific journey possible.

Always Remember:
In Happy moments   Praise God
In Difficult moments Seek God
In Quiet moments   Worship God
In Painful moments Trust God
In Every moment   Thank God!

Table of Contents

Copyright 4

Dedication 6

Introduction: Inspiration 10

Chapter One—My Story 17

Chapter Two—Reinvestment: Embracing Life 26

Chapter Three—Caregiving 32

Chapter Four—Harsh Realities 43

Chapter Five—Demolishing The 'What-Ifs' 52

Chapter Six—The End Of Suffering 59

Chapter Seven—Holding It Together 66

Chapter Eight—Me: A Motherless Daughter 72

Chapter Nine—The Journey Without Mom 78

Chapter Ten—My Love Letter To MOM 88

Acknowledgement 92

About The Author 95

   Ms. Christine Jones M.A. 95

Thank You 99

Notes 101

Introduction: Inspiration

The death of a mother is the first sorrow wept without her.
—Author Unknown

I dedicated my first published poem, "My Mother Inside", to my beautiful, loving mother, Mrs. Gracie Amelina Jones, who died from breast cancer treatments. My poem is written as follows:

"My Mother Inside"
By
Christine Jones

My mother inside smiles at me
My mother inside protects me
My mother inside talks to me
My mother inside visits with me
My mother inside keeps me from harm
My mother inside keeps me warm
My mother inside never leaves me alone
My mother inside is lovely and strong
My mother inside casts a glow of sunshine all through me
My mother inside laughs ever so gently
My mother inside always eases my pain,
And helps prevent me from going insane
My mother inside loves me, for this I know;
She told me this before dying just a few short years ago
My mother inside is virtuous and true
My mother inside is constantly fading,
But always saying, "I LOVE YOU".

Your mom, like mine will always be your best friend. She's the one who kissed you, nurtured you, and cared for you when you were a baby. She eased the pain that comes with being a teen, and helped you as an adult, whether it was helping you make decisions about your personal life, or teaching you how to deal with the ups and downs of being a strong woman. Your mother is and will always be the biggest part of your life. This is a book about dealing with the loss of this strong and beautiful woman and seeking help to deal with the pain and grief that follows. This book is intended to serve women who are religious and who have lost their loving and devoted mothers to cancer, and are ready to go from grief-stricken to full of hope. It will motivate you to find the peace and happiness that you truly deserve, and it will also help you to honor your mom by becoming the strong and happy person she always wanted you to be.

   Throughout the reading of this book, I will show you that I understand your problem, I have love for you because I experienced that exact same problem you are now dealing with, and that you can trust me to help you with this tedious journey, to happiness and peace.

   After twenty-three years without a mother, I am no stranger to searching and loneliness. I can lose myself in reading, journaling, and playing video games for hours at a time. So, when I began writing My

Journey Without Mom, it felt oddly appropriate to spend hours online, in bookstores and libraries searching for books about grief. Those long nights helped me to reflect on the long-term effects of my mother's death. Back then, my family wasn't talking about my mother's death from breast cancer treatments at age seventy-five, and I didn't know anyone in my peer group who mother had died. A book seemed to be a safe and private way to check my feelings against some sort of standard, and I hoped to find one that would help explain what I was feeling—why, in spite of all of my valiant attempts to disassociate myself from the pain and grief of my mother's death, I still miss her twenty-three years later after she died.

In 1995, I became discouraged and dismayed. Despite the plethora of books written about mother-daughter relationships, I found virtually nothing for a woman who'd lost her mother in her thirties. Ten years later I was slightly more successful in my quest. I found self-help books about coping after the loss of a loved one; academic texts about the mourning process in general; psychology books about losing a parent specifically; and narratives by daughters who told their stories of loss, pain, and recovery.

Still, the library shelves didn't address my specific need. Most of these "grief" texts emphasized crisis management over long-term adaptation, failing to acknowledge that part of the adjustment process after the death of a loved one includes, (something that I did not know), maintaining a relationship—albeit a new relationship—with that person. The books I found accurately described the emotional roller coaster we all ride for the first several months after the death of a loved one, but they did not explain how we should, or could, be feeling five, or ten or twenty years after the loss.

I suppose there's a logical reason for this: who, after all, wants to read a book immediately after losing a mother and learn that the mourning process is likely to continue for several decades? We'd all like to believe that mourning is somehow magically contained within those first six months after a loss. I felt horrible enough when my mother died in 1995. I did not want to hear that I'd still miss her in another ten years.

I was in pain and I naturally searched for a quick fix, and I admit that until recently I was no exception. When I began writing My Journey Without Mom, I hoped the two and a half months I planned to devote to this book would provide me with an intense, self-contained period of grief that I could eventually exit and finally, (finally, finally, finally) feel that I didn't long for my mother—or a mother—anymore. But once I began doing research, I realized how unrealistic my expectation was. I discovered that women who had lost their mothers thirty years ago, were still renegotiating their relationships with their mothers and were still missing them and, yes, crying for them, as I still do, today.

More than two decades after my mother's death, I still converse with her. Constantly. I consult her for insights about my father, we argue about his eating habits, and stubbornness, and she urges me to be patient with him. For years this dialogue was my biggest secret, the startling evidence, I was certain, of a daughter whose mourning had gone awry. I discovered that I wasn't the only daughter to grieve this way, and in fact, it is quite normal for a daughter who'd lost her mother. This was a moment of pure joy and relief for me. Thank you, Jesus! For the first time, I felt I didn't have to hide the pain of mother loss; I could accept it as a part of my past and present and get on with enjoying my life.

One of our biggest challenges as adult daughters without mothers is to find a way to see our losses as points of departure rather than dead weights. In this book, you will read the words of a motherless woman who, over the years, have discovered how to use her loss as a catalyst for change, and is trying to embrace and accept that change today.

This is not meant to be a book about how women should mourn. Instead, it's meant to be a book about the variety of ways and techniques used for healthy mourning. And, healthy living.

I wish I had a foolproof plan to offer. I don't. Although this book is structured according to how much time has elapsed since a mother's loss, I don't mean to imply that any kind of rigid schedule exists or should exist. Mourning is a highly individualized process, it's not linear. "It's intensity depends on the age of a daughter when the mother died, the cause of loss, the quality of the mother and daughter relationship, and the support system available both at the time of loss and in subsequent years." Kuber-Ross. Please remember that when a woman is ready to mourn for her mother, she will. Trying to force oneself to take a step before its natural time can be futile as trying to teach a baby to walk.

Chapter One—My Story

> Pain insists upon being attended to. God whispers to us in our pleasures, speaks in our consciences, but shouts in our pains. It is his megaphone to rouse a deaf world.   —C.S. Lewis

I awoke to the covers wrapped so tightly around me. I felt as though I was smothering, but I didn't care. I had never felt so alone in all of my life. I pinched myself, asking out loud to the quiet and stillness of the air in my bedroom, is this real? Can this be actually happening? Did I just bury my mom, a week ago? January 15, 1995 will forever be etched in my brain. My mind was racing, "Why God?" "Why did my sweet and beautiful mother have to get breast cancer and then die from its treatments?" "What the hell just happened?" "What did she do to deserve this?" But most of all, "How do I get through this?" "How do I cope with life after mom?"

For those of you who have lost a loved one, do you ever wonder, did you do all that you were supposed to do to help your loved one while they were alive? I do. Every night before I get into bed, my mom's face appears. I tell her, "I love you, need you and miss you, and I hope that you are happy being with God." I also say, "Mom, please forgive me if I said or did anything to hurt you while you were here with me!"

After my mom's death, I seem to be alive, but not alive. Most of my emotions seemed to have disintegrated, and I was very nervous and anxious all of the time. I felt weak, I could not sleep, and I had very little energy. Do you ever recall feeling this way after your mother's death? But, I also think about the precious moments I shared with my mother. I always give thanks to God for just being alive. During these times, I inhale deeply and very slowly exhale.

Through research, I discovered the Elisabeth Kubler-Ross's model, The Five Stages Of Grief, and I can honestly say that I experienced each and every one of them. They are:

1. **Denial-disbelief about the death of a loved one.**
2. **Anger-anger at your loved one for not taking better care of, or you not taking better care of them.**
3. **Depression-the appropriate response to a great loss. Left in a fog of intense sadness.**
4. **Acceptance-accepting the reality that our loved one is physically gone, for always.**
5. **Bargaining-"what if" and "if only", this had not have happened, then…**

Denial: I am guilty of this! I experienced this before and after my mom's death. Did you? To this very day, I still can't believe the cruel way cancer took my mother's life, her left breast exploding in the bathroom, with skin and blood all over the bathroom sink. Also, the chemo solution which caused her to throw up every day, and the radiation treatments burned her from the inside out, making her skin black as tar. When giving her a bath, she smelled like smoke, I would wipe the burned skin from her body. I always thought that the cancer treatments would cure mom and life would go on as usual. I knew that she was very ill, but no one, not even her doctor told me that she was dying. I was not prepared for losing my mother. It came as a total and complete shock, to me. I said, "God, this not happening to my mother, not my mother!"

Anger: I became a very belligerent, hurt and angry person. Family disappointed me with their lack of empathy. And the reality of it all was, just too much to handle. I knew I had to find a way to deal with my mental stability right then, or I would go insane. Did you experience this, also?

Depression: Hi, I'm Christine, and I was depressed. I have always been a loner. I now know that being alone was the worst possible way to deal with depression. I discovered that I needed help in the worst way. I needed a safe way to release all of the anger, and pain that I was feeling inside. I needed to grieve. I also knew that I had to bring other people into my life to treat my depression. Have you ever been diagnosed with depression?

Acceptance: I did not accept my mom's death until her funeral. It wasn't until I kissed her on her cheek, while she lay in her beautiful pink and white casket. Her skin felt cold and hard to the touch. She also had a tiny smile on the left side of her lips. I called to her, but there was no answer response. There was a stillness and quietness about the funeral chapel and the stinky smell of 'funeral flowers'. Sadly, I realized and accepted, that the woman who had given birth to me was gone forever. Have you truly accepted the death of your mom?

Bargaining: Yup! This was me, also. I used to pray and ask God, "Why did you take my mother away from me?" I would say how sweet and beautiful she was and that she didn't deserve this. I would say take my life and let her come back to be with her loving husband, children and grandchildren. I would say God, "If I never sinned again, would you please bring her back to me?" I realized that God is not a bargainer, and when you try to bargain with him, you always lose. Have you ever bargained with God?

To simply sum up the five stages—it's a very long and painful journey. It's your journey! It's my journey! We all grieve differently. Remember, I love you and this is the unique process I used to help me hug the pain, release, and finally find the peace and happiness that helped me become the person I am today, as a result of losing my mother. It will help you, also.

My brain is well-aware of the fact that my mom is never coming back, but twenty-three years later, it seems like my heart refuses to accept her absence. I still have the same dream each night. I envision her in that same cream-colored three-piece outfit she wore in her casket, during her funeral. Her black hair was cut in a short afro, thin eyebrows, and smooth brown lips. She looked as if Heaven itself had laid her there in front of me. Yet in the midst of this tranquility, misery was present. There was a handsome looking fair skinned man with reddish brown hair who looked spiffy in his three-piece black suit and hat. He looked as if he was attending a wedding. But instead of tears of joy, his voice resounded in shrills of agonizing sobs. He looked as if he lost control of his body, haunching over with his head down in his hands. He was clearly not getting married, yet the phrase "till death do us part" had its place in the matter. "Do us part" was now. That man was my mother's husband. And that man is my father.

My mom's funeral took place on January 15, 1995 in Hayti, Missouri. I was thirty-three years old at the time. But sometimes, no matter how hard you try to hold on to the pain, the reality is that in this life we all have our breaking point, and if you do not find a safe way to release the pain, you will shut down. And so, when no one was around, I fell apart, by screaming, crying, and cursing. I eventually turned to writing as a way of releasing my pain. I wrote about being angry with my mother for dying, the precious memories that she and I shared, and how cancer ravaged her body, and took her life. Those memories marked the beginning of a unending love affair with the written word. Looking back, I realized that my mom's death gave birth to my passion for writing.

Coping with loss

Here are some strategies I used to help me cope with the loss of my mother and move forward.

1. I always talk about my mother. I never leave her out of any discussions. Talking about her and memories of her helps me to release the pain and find peace. Remember, denying that her death occurred will isolate and frustrate you to the point where you might become a danger to yourself.
2. Welcome your feelings about you mother's death. Whether it is sadness, anger, frustration, and even exhaustion, remember the feelings are all normal.
3. Eat healthy, exercise and get as much rest as possible will help you move forward, day by day.
4. Do you want to feel better? Then, reach out to others who have experienced a loss like yours.
5. Do something in memory of your mother. For example, plant a tree, participate in a walkathon, or throw a party to celebrate her life.

The takeaway points that I hope you got from the chapter is first and foremost is that with the five stages of grief comes the knowledge of grief's terrain, making us better equipped to cope with life and loss. We all grieve differently. And, in order to deal with your mom's death you

MUST allow yourself time to grieve first and then deal with the loss, by using the strategies mentioned above.

Chapter Two—Reinvestment: Embracing Life

Everything is irrelevant but this: embrace life. To feel it. To savor it. To love it.
—Mary Rubin

My story was all about how you and I are alike; losing our mothers from cancer and coping with the grief and loss that followed. It also helped me to reinvest in my future and embrace life again.

According to Ashley Davis Prend, A.C.S.W., in her book, "Transcending Loss", "Reinvestment is a broad term to describe the phenomenon of connecting with life again, of caring enough to dedicate yourself to the living and to the future. But it's not just that you return to work or that you go back to your "old" life. You are forever changed. You cannot just go back to life as if nothing has happened, because something has happened, and life will never be the same. So, Reinvestment really means accepting the loss and channeling your pain, creating something meaningful that is a direct result of your experience with loss.

There are many different ways of reinvesting. Some reinvest in love, others in a creative project. Some reinvest in a new career, others in a new cause or mission. You see, when your loved one was alive, you invested a certain amount of energy into your relationship with that person. When she died, you spent a certain amount of energy grieving and mourning her. In Transcendence, you take that same energy and you channel it into something productive, something meaningful, something full of life.

Reinvestment is, in many ways, the ultimate expression of human resilience, the consummate triumph of the human spirit. Reinvestment means that even when loss tramples your heart and shatters your spirit, it is possible that you like a mythical bird, the phoenix, can rise from the ashes to embrace life anew. Grievers who choose to do this are reaffirming their rightful place in a world where life, love, loss, and death coexist.

Reinvestment in Love

If we invest in love again we may lose again. A common defense is to protect ourselves from the possibility of future losses by barricading our broken hearts. Certainly, this desire is understandable and perhaps even necessary, initially. But over time those who keep their hearts guarded under lock and key may protect themselves from pain, but they also prevent any real joy from touching their lives. The bottom line is if you don't risk, you don't love. And without love, life can be very hollow indeed.

Loss, unfortunately, can stifle the ability to love. Although all losses are painful, and many factors contribute to make each loss personally unique and meaningful to each griever, the loss of a child is generally recognized as the most severe, the most wretched, the most awful.

But how do you make yourself love again when you know that the price for love is the potential for loss? Well, it's not easy. It's a process of working through the feelings; it takes time. First you have to do the grief work, because otherwise you're really not in a position to give. The reality is that few people can or do reinvest in love so quickly without first going through the deep grieving process. Of course there are exceptions to every rule, but in general, time to grieve is required before a person should reinvest in love.

If you "love" again too quickly, it may be a way of avoiding the pain of the grief work. Jumping back into relationships before you've grieved is not the answer. You cannot replace that which was lost. Sooner or later, one way or another, the grief must be confronted, felt and processed.

Transcending reinvestment in love does not try to replace. It recognizes the loss and accepts the changes as part of the reality of living and losing. Transcending reinvestment in love, is a process of integrating the old with the new.

For some, the future after the loss of a loved one seems impossible. And they can't imagine loving again. All their emotional energy is tied up in grief and anguish; they have nothing left to give anyone else. But as difficult as it is, if we allow ourselves to reinvest, to reconnect with other people, we can begin healing and move toward Transcendence.

Reinvestment over Time

Some grievers will choose to always be involved with causes that are related to their grief. Other grievers will do it for a time and then later move on to other projects. Transcendence is fluid and reinvestments change over time. And their goals and purposes change over time. Sometimes they are motivated by the desire to help others, and at other times, they are motivated by the need to help self. But what is consistent and critical in defining and understanding reinvestments as a means to Transcendence, is that they are about channeling the pain and energy stimulated by the loss into something meaningful and productive."

It is my hope that your takeaway from this chapter is that knowing that although life will never be the same, with using the techniques mentioned, you will experience a positive change in a positive way. These techniques build a bridge back to life—a different life, to be sure—but life nevertheless.

Chapter Three—Caregiving

> Grief is a reaction to a loss, but it can be—and with caregivers' grief often is—a multifaceted reaction.
> —Kenneth Dora, PhD

Caring for my mother during her illness was one way that I was able to find new ways to reinvest in myself and embrace my future. Although I endured heart wrenching pain while caring for her, it also allowed me to be happy at times, and focus on a future without her. I thoroughly enjoyed pampering my mom and keeping her happy during this terrible time in her life. By taking care of her, I was inadvertently taking care of myself, and my well-being.

As a former home caregiver to my mother, I experienced a profound sense of loss, and I went through a period of denial, after her death. The grief I experienced triggered mixed emotions, and I was faced with a barrage of conflicting feelings. I realized that I had begun grieving before my mother's death. During the course of her chronic, illness, I experienced a range of emotions such as: hopelessness, stress, and guilt. After her death, I experienced sadness, anger and depression. As a home caregiver, it important to acknowledge this grief. I didn't. The job was very stressful and tiring to me, and according to Michael Schreiner, in Gestalt psychology "unacknowledged grief is unable or unwilling to move through the needs satisfaction cycle in order to close an open gestalt." My doctor also told me that not acknowledging grief and loss can build up to caregiver burnout.

Here are ways that you can work through the barrage of emotions, that you may be feeling after your mother's death and regain some normalcy in your life:

- Were you ever a caregiver to your mom? I was. Did you experience burnout while taking care of her? I did. To help with caregiver burnout, get involved in various community activities— such as before and after school tutoring. Set up regular "me time" for yourself. Make sure that you are not socially isolated. Go to the gym, ride a bike, go to the salon and get your hair and nails done. And treat yourself by going to your favorite restaurant.
- As a caregiver, do not hesitate to seek help for yourself if needed. I did. And, this was a bad mistake. Find and write down the names of people who could be a strong part of your network, such as family members, friends, a love interest, church members, and neighbors.

- Next, in order to use your network effectively, create a list of assigned tasks to various people. Here is how it is written:

SL (sincere listeners):	Ds (doers):	R&R (rest and relaxation):
_____	_____	_____
_____	_____	_____
_____	_____	_____
_____	_____	_____

- Do you have a remaining parent who is alive and well? If so, hire a caregiver to take care of this parent, see to their needs, and do routine chores such as laundry and cleaning. This will relieve burn-out and allow more time for yourself.
- Always take very good care of yourself. Do not miss doctor appointments. I missed several doctor appointments with my ophthalmologist. I did not take my eye medicine as prescribed, didn't get my eye pressures checked regularly, and ended up developing glaucoma. This is a disease that I will have for the rest of my life. Do not let this happen to you! If someone dies and you

are the caregiver, be mindful of your eating, sleeping, and exercise habits. "This is where the me time becomes especially important."

Remember, after the death of a loved one it is easy to ignore that a horrific lost has occurred in the family. Give yourself time to grieve about the changes that have happened in your life. When you can do this, your feelings will less often erupt as angry outbursts weighed down by guilt, or creep over you as depression and hopelessness. They will instead become more easily expressed as a shared loss of something treasured—which family and friends close to the situation can likely empathize with, leading to a deeper communication and stronger relationships with those going through the loss with you.

Next, did you have to deal with the denial that came after your mother's death? If you did you discovered that denial is a coping mechanism that gives you time to adjust to distressing situations—but staying in denial can help and it can also hurt, and allow grief, depression and other emotions to spiral out of control. Stop denying your mother's death and say," My mother is dead, and she is never coming back to me!" The release from grief and pain will be monumental! It will be astounding! The horrendous burden of grief and pain will be lifted finally, and you will move forward with your life.

Did you know that refusing to acknowledge that something is wrong is a way of coping with emotional conflict, stress, painful thoughts, and anxiety? Did you do this after your mother's death? Where you in deep denial back then, that you would not acknowledge the fact that your mother was gone forever? Was it hard for you to face the fact that you had to continue life's journey without your mother, and that you would never see, feel or touch her again? Did you totally shut down?

I experienced all of the emotions mentioned above, and I finally reached to my doctor for help. She completely turned me around with what she had to say. Dr. Rieker said that, "Denial can be very helpful, and harmful if allowed to continue for too long. Refusing to face facts might seem unhealthy. Sometimes, though, a short period of denial can be helpful. Being in denial gives your mind the opportunity to unconsciously absorb shocking or distressing information, like your mother's death, at a pace that you can handle. Therefore, by initially denying your mother's death, you are allowing your mind time to adsorb the possibility of it and therefore, will eventually accept the loss more rationally." She also said to seek more professionally help, if needed.

Here are some steps to recovery that I used to help me deal more effectively with the loss, grief, pain and denial of my mother's death. According to Bob Deits, in his book, "Life After Loss", there are four steps to walking the path to wholeness. They are:

- Shock and numbness
- Denial and withdrawal
- Acknowledgement and pain
- Adaptation and renewal

1. Shock and Numbness

"In the first seven to ten days after a major loss you will probably be stunned, shocked and overwhelmed. You may feel "frozen" or hysterical. Either way, you will have a difficult time later remembering much of what took place.

Whatever your initial outward reaction, you will have a certain numbness inside. Your emotional system has shut down for the time being. I like to think of it as God or nature supplying us with temporary protection against the full impact of our losses. The experience of shock provides us with a brief, sheltered rest before we begin the long journey through grief, then the agony of grief toward a renewed sense of joy.

A few days after the death of a loved one, when the funeral is over and relatives have gone home, the shock begins to wear off. This is a good time to have someone with you. It is a poor time to make decisions that will have a lasting impact on your life.

Shock follows every loss experience to some degree. The important things for you to know about shock are:

- It is a necessary first step to recovery.
- It doesn't last long.
- It is not a time for long-term decision making.
- It is good to have a trusted friend with you.
- When shock goes away pain arrives."

2. Denial and Withdrawal

"When the shock or your loss wears off, you will want to deny what has happened with all, your strength.

As unavoidable and natural as loss is, we are seldom ready to admit that loss is a normal part of our own life. We seldom stop to think that our parents will die someday—that the loss will occur in our lifetime.

It's natural to deny a loss when to acknowledge it leads to so much pain. Physical and emotional affects you may experience after the initial shock wears off include:

- Feeling weak and drained of energy
- Inability to perform routine tasks
- Lack of appetite
- Lack of sleep or oversleeping
- Lack of concern with personal hygiene or grooming
- Fantasies of the deceased person
- Expecting a dead person to come back
- Anger

These are all normal reactions to loss and if you know to expect these signs of denial and withdrawal after a loss, you can comfort yourself by saying, "This reaction is normal. This is another step on the way through grief. I will not always feel like this."

3. **Acknowledgement and Pain**

"Acknowledging a loss is the most important step of your recovery. It is at this point that you will again take full charge of your life and full responsibility for your feelings. A noticeable sense of balance is coming back into your life when you can acknowledge that your loss is real—and permanent. It represents a giant step toward full recovery.

You will be tempted to slip back into denial of what has happened. You can do that periodically and you will feel better—for a little while. But the only pathway to balance and wholeness lies through the pain of acknowledgement of your loss.

The acknowledgement phase is a long one, and for that reason it is extremely important that you have a strong support system in place as you find your way through it. This is an up-and-down phase. You will not stay immersed in agony for a year and then suddenly wake up one morning to find yourself finished with it. You will make progress one day and encounter difficulties the next, but overall you will be heading in the right direction. Those who have been there assure the rest of us that slowly but surely, the good days begin to outnumber the bad ones."

4. **Adaptation and renewal**

"The first sign that the roughest part or your grief is over will be when you notice a change in the questions you ask yourself. From the time of your loss, the most haunting. And a persistent question is, "Why did this happen to me?" The day will come, often a year or more after the loss, when a new question will emerge. That question is, "How can I grow through this tragic event to become a better person?"

When you stop asking "why?" And begin asking "how?" You are beginning to adapt to your new life without the person, place or condition that has been lost. You will emerge as a new person in your own right."

It is my hope that from this chapter you gained insight on how caregiving can get you to happy and that by recognizing the steps to recovery, you will walk the path to wholeness, and successfully journey forward to happiness and peace.

Chapter Four—Harsh Realities

You are drawing out things in your life that are of a similar vibration to what you are thinking and feeling.
—Law of Attraction

Caregiving allowed me to spend time with and bond with my ailing mother. It also allowed me to take care of her as she took care of me as a baby. Although I loved taking care of my mom, it was very stressful at times, and it took every ounce of my energy to do so. Being positive and focused help me to stay the course.

Most people are not aware that if they changed their primary thoughts to positive ones, they would actually be able to change their lives for the better and find peace and happiness. Instead they tend to focus on "what is or what they do not want", instead of what they truly desire. Unfortunately, by focusing in this way, the world, itself, continues to bring more things into their lives with the same equilibrium of these negative thoughts.

The bottom line is that in order for you to heal after a loss, you must at least attempt to focus more on the positive and happy aspects around you. This isn't always easy, especially after the death of a loved one! However, it is important to understand that your main thoughts are creating the dominant feelings you are having, not the other way around. So doesn't it make sense to say that when you carefully change your thoughts from negative ones to positive ones, you will begin to feel better as well?

But how can you focus on the positive and not focus on "what is" as you are going through the grieving process? Here are some small, but very significant steps you can take to help you to change your thoughts and feel better at this very difficult time.

1. How are you feeling?

The first step is to notice how you're feeling. If you're feeling badly, chances are you're thinking negative thoughts. If you are feeling happy, you are probably thinking good thoughts. The more powerful your thoughts are, whether they are good or bad, the more they will affect your feelings. I discovered that when I am thinking about something negative, like how the cancer destroyed my mother's body, I am feeling depressed. I quickly remember that she is with God and is okay. I start to feel happy again.

2. The "Yes, But" Game.

Again, the key is to deliberately try to think more powerful, positive thoughts, try playing the "Yes, But" game. I always say, "Yes," "But mom is with me always with me". "That is, after you think a negative thought, follow it with, "Yes, but," and add a statement of something good that came out of it. For example, you may be thinking of how much you miss your loved one. Then follow that thought with, "Yes, but we had a wonderful and beautiful life together." And then continue with even more positive thoughts, such as, "I am so grateful that my mom was in my life." If you can, follow that with some funny memories you shared with your loved one. Then continue to think of more and more positive aspects and memories. In this way, you will be focusing on your love and the good times you had with your loved one, instead of the absence of her." — Unknown Author

3. Feeling better.

Speak to others about the good times you and your loved enjoyed together. You will be so surprised how this helps you to feel better. You are thinking about her anyway, so express those great thoughts to your listener. I used to talk about how mom would straighten my hair with a pressing comb. It did not take very long for her to do because I have very soft hair. Mom would always burn my right ear with the pressing comb. It seems like it took years for the feeling to come back to the tip of that ear! (Hallelujah! Thank God for permed and natural hair styles).

4. Let your loved one be your guide.

Now for the big surprise! Ask your loved one for guidance as you plan on what to do next, in your life. Then make sure to listen to your gut feelings and act upon them, quickly. You should receive answers and wonderful words of wisdom that comes as thoughts and feelings. When I was considering retiring from teaching, I asked my mom, "Mom, should I retire, should I just give it up and walk away, after thirty years?" A resounding "Yes", entered my thoughts. And then this thought entered my mind, after you retire you will have the time to pursue your dream to become a published author. I listened, and I prayed, and now my dream to be a published author has come true.

5. The right vibe.

Focus on finding the right people with the right vibe that will help you to heal. You will see how the universe will then work in ways to make that happen! They may show up in your life unexpectedly; friends and relatives may talk about those who have helped them; you may read about local people on the internet who help others to heal; the list can go on and on. And since you are religious, talk to your minister. I talked to my pastor, it really, really helped me, and it will help you. Just make sure to pay attention to all those who are coming into your awareness. Then, trust your instincts about whether or not those people will be able to help you.

6. Pray.

Always pray! Ask God and his angels to help you. When you pray, expect the help that you are seeking. Instead of begging God, thank him, even before your prayer has been answered. For example, say, "Thank you so much for helping me to feel better." In other words, have complete faith that your prayer is going to be answered now—not some later in your life!

7. Meditate.

Meditate! Participate! Praying is talking to God, but meditating is listening to him. As in any relationship, it is important to listen as well as speak. When you quiet your thoughts and meditate, you are focused and is in a better position to feel a connection with God, the angels and your deceased loved one. I tried meditating after speaking with my doctor, shortly after my mother died. It worked. I did feel a closer connection to my mom. It worked for me. It will work for you. Happy Meditating!

8. Make positive declarations.

Repeat positive declarations throughout the day. Make sure they are stated in the present tense and you feel at peace when you say them. Some examples are: it is okay for me to heal; I am able to feel my loved one whenever I choose. I always receive signs and messages from my loved one. I choose to feel better today. It is good for me to pamper myself as I heal. I discover new strengths that I did not know I had, every day; God is healing my heart more and more each day; and I will be happy and find peace again. Making positive declarations, will help you feel positive about life's journey ahead.

9. Harmony.

Try to maintain a mutual harmony in all of your relationships and in the situations around you. Make a point of being with those who lift your spirit and refrain from doing anything that you cannot handle, yourself. Leave all of the naysayers behind. Surround yourself with positive people, and those who have experienced the situation you are now in.

10. Have a fun day out.

Treat yourself to something fun and do anything that makes you happy. Sometimes that may mean just going to the mall, going for a walk, listening to your favorite music, going out with friends, sitting quietly, reading a book, writing, or anything else that puts you in a better feeling place. I do all of these things occasionally, when I have time. Try them, they really do work.

11. Release the grief and find peace.

Have an attitude of, today I am going to release the grief and find peace. Really take notice of all of the good things in your life each day. If you have the time, sit down and write a list of all of your blessings. Then, whenever you begin to feel sad, make sure to take out that list and redirect your attention to these positive aspects once again. What will your list include? The number one person on my list who I am blessed to have in my life is my one-hundred-year-old dad, who lives with me, and who I adore.

For you to feel better, it is very important that you begin to focus on how happy your deceased loved one was before she died, not how they died, but, on the blessings in your life, on the happy times, on the things you love, and on positive goals ahead of you. At first it may seem like a daunting task, given all that has happened, but after a while of deliberately changing your thoughts to more positive ones, it will get easier and easier. Writing down your blessings, goals and memories is a great way to start. Repeating positive declarations throughout the day also helps immensely. It doesn't matter how you choose to do it. Just make the choice to feel better and be happier! According to the Law of Attraction, you get what you think about most of the time. So, it makes sense to begin to focus on more positive, loving thoughts throughout each day. Remember, if you make the necessary changes to your life mentioned above, you will like I did, release the grief and find peace and therefore find happiness.

Chapter Five—Demolishing The 'What-Ifs'

Don't let the what-ifs or should haves hold you back! It is your time and your dreams.
—Unknown Author

Even though I have had to face some harsh realities since the death of my mother, I have tried to live my life with the least number of what-ifs as possible. By doing this I have been able to move forward, instead of wondering what if this had happened, or what if that had happened. This helps me get rid of the clutter and have clear thoughts in my mind.

On January 8. 1995, my mother took her final breath. After years of suffering, my mother was no longer in pain, and her body was no longer betraying her. That moment was one of the most shocking and heartbreaking events in my life. The period that followed was full of confusing and turbulent events.

The role of caregiver to my mother became a part of me. It became a part of my psyche and I identified with it. I helped my mom with her medicine regimen, attended doctor appointments with her, prepared her meals, gave her baths and so on. So, what was I supposed to do now that my caregiver role had come to a halt?

With my caregiver journey ending, I was beginning a new journey—one of grieving, healing and try to find what my "new normal" would be. What would it be like without an adrenaline rush whenever the phone would ring, after mom was admitted to the hospital that final time? What would it be like without Mom—no mother to call when I needed my "Mom", and no mother needing me? Would I be okay without being needed? I do not know!

This identity crisis was quickly followed by "what-ifs" and "should-haves": What if I had done a better job at paying closer attention to her? What if my dad and mom had chosen a better treatment option? I should have taken off work to go to the doctor with her and discussed cancer treatments in depth! What if I had talked to her more about dipping snuff, and the dangers involved? What if she had not breast-fed me? What if she had not lived in a house where smoking was permitted and tolerated? The truth is, I did the best job that I knew how, by giving my mother 110 percent of my effort, time and attention. I simply was making myself suffer with 20/20 hindsight.

This January 15, it will be twenty-four years since my mom passed away. Not a day goes by without my thinking of her. With each passing day, however, the ability to cope gets a little bit easier. The void in my heart fills with memories of love, not loss; the pit in my stomach aches less, now; and my outlook on the future is that I will have loads and loads of happiness and peace. My experience most certainly has defined me. I did not, however, let it destroy me. I chose to draw from it as a way of bringing comfort and guidance to myself and you, who is now in this stage of the journey. It is to you that I have this to say about losing your loved one:

1. Have compassion for yourself.

Do not let the what-ifs and should-haves define you. In other words, don't let them still your joy. It is important to always remember that you became a caregiver because you care. You stepped up, took charge, and gave the situation your all. The outcome may not have been the outcome you hoped for, bargained for, or wished for on a shooting star, but it is your new reality. Cut yourself some slack; do not ponder over the should have, could have, would have, and what-ifs. Be kind to yourself and to others; forgive yourself for anything that you feel you could have done better or more of; and know the person you cared for was loved and respected and felt loved, throughout the entire terrible ordeal. Do not feel guilty about not doing enough. You did all you could have possibly done to keep your mom healthy and happy.

2. Life goes on

Following my mother's death, I was convinced that there was absolutely, positively no way that life could go on. In my opinion, the world tilted on it axis that January 15, 1995. But as much as I felt that the world had come to a screeching halt for all of humanity, life in fact continued on normally for everyone but my family. And so it will be with you. I was introduced to the "thirty day" rule by a doctor of mine. It goes as follows: the first 30 days after a loss or a catastrophe, the phone may ring, the mailbox may be full of cards and the refrigerator may be stocked full of fried chicken from your closest friends. Very quickly though, life moves on for those not directly involved. At that time, begin seeking help from those who bring you comfort on a regular basis—be it a sibling, best friend, or extended family member. If your confidante happens to be the loved one who died be sure to find a support group who can help you transition. Life goes on whether you want it to or not. How you handle the transition will determine if you find happiness or remain in the valley of sadness. I choose happiness for you.

3. Do not make any drastic "what-ifs" decisions.

Here is the best piece of advice I received, from a friend who had lost her mom when she was my age: "Give yourself two years. Something changed for me at that time. My brain fog cleared, the hurt subsided, and I felt better about making changes." While the two-year mark turned out to be spot on for her, it was not that way with me. It took me much longer. It may not be the transformation landmark for you either. Regardless, take the time to do some healing and traveling before you decide to take all of loved one's possessions to a thrift store or sell your home and move to another state (as I wanted to do). Take your time and make the right decisions. All you have is time. There is no need to rush.

4. Allow yourself the grieving and processing time.

Any wound, physical or emotional, requires time to heal. Remember everybody grieves differently, but as a general rule, you will have good days and not so-good days. Give yourself permission to cry when you feel like crying; excuse yourself from situations that trigger you; and simply do not answer the phone or get on Facebook if you are not up for yet another heart-to-heart with yet another concerned individual. This time is yours! Do not let anyone steal it from you!

Get rid of your what-ifs, and you will feel lighter and happier and probably more fulfilled and certain of what you really want in life. Please remember that the "what-ifs" and "should-haves" are designed to hug the grief and pain and not release it. It is my hope for you that you will have the happiness and the peace that you deserve after you have demolished, or gotten rid of the "what-ifs" and "should-haves" by using the process mentioned in this chapter. It is my promise to you that will get and maintain the peaceful and happy life you have always wanted.

Chapter Six—The End Of Suffering

We have to confront ourselves. Do we like what we see in the mirror? And, according to our light, according to our understanding, according to our courage, we will have to say yea or nay—and rise!
—Maya Angelou

I realized that I could not become who I needed to become by remaining who I was. After the death of my mother, I became very depressed. I had low self-esteem. I was dissatisfied with things about me, and therefore, I was dissatisfied with certain things about other people.

There was also a time after my mom's death that I wanted to check out of life. I was not sure that I could face the future without her. I knew for certain that I could not face the pain of not having her around anymore. Suicide was on my mind and in my thoughts, constantly. Anxiety was taking control of me and I could not stop it. I was turning into someone I did not recognize. I stayed in my house a lot during this dark period. It felt as if my world was shrinking by leaps and bounds. Then finally, and very slowly, I made the decision to stand up and fight. And fight I did. I fought for life. I fought for happiness. I fought for peace. I did not want to die, but I did not know how to live, without mom. I finally realized that although losing my mother was very painful, I had consciously made the choice to suffer. The question now was, how was I going to end the suffering?

So, I decided to work on becoming a better, happier, and a more likable me. I did not like who I had become, and I wanted to change that. I hated me and anything about me. After all, it is quite miserable to live a life being depressed all the time. They say that misery loves company, but I think the company that misery attracts is terrible by nature. It only makes you unhappy and unhealthy, and then before you know it, you have turned into an illusion of your former self.

At present, I am almost pleased with who I am. I can't say that I am perfect or that I have achieved my ideal self, because there is still so much I have to work on. I also believe that becoming a better person is something that I will be working on, for a long time. But I have started on this journey, the journey of life.

In this chapter I share with you the process I used for becoming a better person, and finding the good things in life, again. It is about becoming someone you truly love and adore, which will then bring peace and happiness into your life. If you have been feeling stuck, where you are in life, right now, these ideas will help you find the peace, happiness and inspiration to move forward:

1. Allow yourself to become the person you were always meant to be, by experiencing life and living it to the fullest.
2. Work on any of your personal qualities that may prevent you from becoming the happy person you want to be.
3. Become more involved in community activities.
4. Treat others the way you want to be treated.
5. Take college courses to equip yourself with the skills needed to become the new you.
6. Make allowances for differences in other people's attitudes, and opinions.
7. Be ready for positive change when it comes.
8. Formulate new everyday routines; change is always good.
9. If possible, visit other countries and cultures to become more of a well -rounded individual.
10. Be considerate of others.
11. Do something that produces change; a walkathon for cancer perhaps!

12. Do not let fear resonate in your mindset.

13. Be approachable.

14. Dream big, think big!

15. Serve with a compassionate heart.

16. Always entertain positive thoughts.

I also use music as inspiration for my life. My all- time favorite actress, singer and performer is Whitney Houston. When I am down and feeling low I listen to her song, 'I Look To You'. it inspires me to have daily talks about depression, and peace with God, who is my constant companion and stress reliever. I especially like these lyrics from her song, "I Look To You":

> As I lay me down
> Heaven hear me now
> I'm lost without a cause
> After giving it my all
> Winter storms have come
> And darkened my sun
> After all that I've been through
> Who on earth can I turn to?
> I look to you,
> I look to you
> After all my strength is gone
> In you I can be strong
> I look to you,
> I look to you, yea
> And when melodies are gone

In you I hear a song
I look to you, you
About to lose my breath
There's no more fighting left
Sinking to rise no more
Searching for that open door
And every road that I've taken, mmm
Led to my regret
And I don't know if I'm going to make it
Nothing to do but lift my head
I look to you,
I look to you, yea
And when all my strength is gone
In you I can be strong
I look to you.

One of my favorite books of all time that inspired me to make positive changes in my life is Getting To Happy by Terry McMillan. This book changed and blessed my soul!!!! Thank you God!!!! The message I got from this book is about love and friendship. Loving yourself and others unselfishly, the importance of friendship, and chasing the perennial goal-getting to happy, are the themes of this book. My favorite inspirational movie is "Lean On Me". This movie is about asking for help when you need it.

FYI: I also became a Christian many years ago and discovered that I truly found peace and happiness in doing what I love to do and that is serving my lord and savior, Jesus Christ.

It is my goal for you to listen to Whitney Houston's song, "I Look To You", and to read Terry McMillan's book, 'Getting To Happy', for inspiration to end your suffering and grief. Doing this will help you move forward in life and find happiness and peace.

Chapter Seven—Holding It Together

Challenges make you discover things about yourself that you never really knew.
—Cicely Tyson

As my grief and suffering comes to an end, I begin to experience challenges, that will make me a stronger person. Grief, just like cancer is a disease of this century. No one will escape its presence. You can compare it to the weather. When rain is predicted in the forecast, it's not just for a certain group of people. Everyone will experience it during their lifetime. Some people will be more prepared to handle it than others. It is important that you realize that everyone handles grief differently, If you prepare for life's stressors, such as grief, pain, and depression, then you will get soaked, but not drown. If you are not prepared for life's stressors, then you will drown under their weight. I discovered that my stressors were too great and too many for me to handle in my own strength, and that peace was still possible if I prayed and did things God's way.

Do not be scared to make the necessary changes that God may tell you to make to leave grief's highway. His way will be better and much easier than your way. Hear what the Holy Spirit is saying to you. Remember you control your destiny. Every event in your life reflects a decision you made. So make the best possible decisions when it comes to your life.

Holding it together after a loved one has died takes quite a toll. It may take many years before you get back the normalcy you once had in your life. But do not despair, when God is called upon, he will show up and he will show out, in your life. Pray and keep praying. Be honest about your stressors and do not try to rationalize them away. Know when you are being your own worst enemy and are destroying your own peace.

Life is not always easy to deal with. Accidents happen, businesses fail and loved ones pass on. When my world fell apart, it was very difficult for me to keep myself intact. Believe me, I have been there!

After the death of my mother, I almost lost my ability to teach school. I began to develop a love-hate relationship with my students. At that time, I did not particularly care for some of the people I worked around, and I would take days off from work sporadically, just to be free from it all. And, I really did not want to be a teacher anymore. I very nearly came undone. But, I still had an elderly father and a sick brother to take care of and provide for. I had bills to pay, and I had no choice but to carry on.

Finding acceptance is the key to keeping it together. According to Elisabeth Kubler-Ross, "Finding acceptance may be just having more good days than bad. As we begin to live again and enjoy our life, we often feel that in doing so, we are betraying our loved one. We can never replace what has been lost, but we can make new connections, new meaningful relationships, new interdependencies. Instead of denying our feelings, we listen to our needs; we move, we change, we grow, we evolve. We may start to reach out to others and become involved in their lives. We invest in our friendships and in our relationship with ourselves. We begin to live again, but we cannot do so until we have given grief its time."

Keeping it together when you want to fall apart is not easy. I am living proof that it is possible! And in the end, it is worth it!

Here are seven helpful tips that you can integrate into your life, to help you to hold it together, when times get tough:

1. Focus on the present and what matters the most. Forget about the notion that being busy means one is accomplishing things of importance. Look at your day to day activities and prioritize your

tasks. Do the pressing tasks today and save the others for another day. Change what you can and leave the rest to God!

2. Talking to a family member, a trusted friend, or a counselor about your grief is a good way to release it. Sharing thoughts will help you to release the internal pressure buildup and gain a new perspective, from other people about the situation. Remember, a shared problem is a problem divided between two people, to take the pressure off of one!

3. Talk to someone who has gone through the same situation as you, and if you are strong enough, follow that advice yourself. Your own advice is relevant and important to your own well-being.

4. One way that you can release negativity when you are alone and in a safe place, is to scream, and then scream some more. Other ways include talking to God, and journaling. Negativity can fester, therefore, do whatever it takes to get rid of it!

5. Always be grateful. Focusing on the people and things in your life that you are grateful and love for improves your attitude, thereby improving your health. Showing gratitude leads to a positive attitude.

6. Live, love and laugh. Live for the future! Love forever! Laugh always! Laugh at life, laugh at yourself! Find the positive in every situation. Remember, to do you!
7. Be patient and surround yourself with a strong network of family, friends, and loved ones. Remember, prayer is always the answer. Prayer changes the person and the situation that is being prayed about.

My hope for you is that after you have used the helpful tips given here you will hold it together and leave grief's highway. Your stressors will be gone, and you will be able to move forward into a happy and fulfilled life.

Chapter Eight—Me: A Motherless Daughter

> When a mother dies, a daughter grieves. And then her life moves on. She does thankfully, feel happiness again. But the missing her, the wanting her, the wishing she were still here—I will not lie to you, although you probably know. That part never ends.
> —Hope Edelman

After trying to hold it together for more than twenty years since the death of my mother, I have gained a deeper level of reflection and awareness. I have had plenty of time not only to think about the long-term effects of mother loss, but also the influence it has had on my life. And, I have also found that according to Taranjit K. Bhakti, PsyD, "Research tends to overlook adult women who lose their moms, because they're already adults, people assume these daughters don't need maternal guidance." I needed maternal guidance then, and I still do now. Do you?

Although my mother died twenty-three years ago, I still think of her every day, with deep longing triggered by very specific joyful and painful events. I am still surprised by the intensity of the grief during these times. I discovered that subsequent losses in particular, such as the thought of my brother's death, always sends me back to mourning my mother, and evoking the same emotions and fears I had when my mother died. It is important for you and I to remember that mourning can only be resolved to the best of our ability, in any particular time in our life. That is why I felt that I had worked through my grief for my mother at age thirty-three, but now I find myself facing additional challenges at age fifty-five which has forced me to rework the loss from my slightly altered perspective.

A significant transformation has occurred in me and it has in you also, that our longing for our mothers, continues to recede further into the past, has been replaced by a more generalized longing for a mother. Adult motherless, Christian daughters such as you and I, haven't and probably never will lose the need or the desire for such a figure in our lives.

The closer I get to the Magic Number, for me it is seventy-five, that is the age when my mother died, I live with the fear that my life will be cut short, as my mother's was. I have the desire to cram in as much as I can before reaching age seventy—the year of mother's cancer diagnosis and mastectomy. So, what do I do? What do you do? Travel, get married, write a number one best- selling novel, go mountain climbing…Some people think I am crazy. They just don't understand that if I don't meet certain challenges now, there might not be enough time to experience the thrill of these activities later.

For me, reaching the Magic Number triggers a grief response. It is a time of both sadness and rebirth. Sadness in that I am doing things that my mother never got to do, such as traveling to Washington D.C., and becoming a published author, and feeling relieved that my destiny will differ from my mom's.

There are other things that I would like to share about myself that puts me back into the throes of grief, sometimes. I can no longer hear my mother's voice. Have you experienced this? This one really gets to me. I can't remember the sound of my mother's voice. This was lost to me within three to four years after she died. I regret that I did not think to get her voice on tape. But I believe that if she were to call me on the phone from the beyond, I would immediately recognize her voice after twenty-three years.

With each new challenge that I have had to face, I have been frightened to do so without my mother's support. I have reached out to my mother but, of course, she wasn't there. The last milestone I had with my mother was turning thirty, which happened three years before her death. I was depressed because most of my friends were married and I wasn't. Although she was gravely ill, she comforted me, and said it would be alright. She said it will happen when it is supposed to.

But some of the worst feelings surrounding milestones comes with the ones never reached. There is one in particular that I will be mentioned. I sometimes am glad my mother did not get to see me at age fifty-five, unmarried and childless.

I was also clingy. I did not want to get rid of or give away any of my mother's possessions after she died. I kept everything exactly the way she left it. Years later my dad and I realized this was foolish and allowed family members to get some of mom's things and we donated the rest. I still have her gold wedding bands, as a keepsake.

Because I am the "baby" of the family, I thought it gave me certain privileges. I was very selfish at times and I did not want to share my parents with any of my other siblings. My dad and mom spoiled me and I felt as though I was their only child. They doted on me, and I felt very special and proud to be their baby girl. I was protected and loved, and I still feel protected and loved by mom, today. I hope this is a feeling that I share with you. My wish for you is that you are loved and still feel the protection of your mother, with you and around you, each day.

Chapter Nine—The Journey Without Mom

"If Roses Grow In Heaven"
"If roses grow in Heaven
Lord, pick a bunch for me,
Place them in my mother's arms
And tell her they're from me.
Tell her I love and miss her,
And when she turns to smile,
Place a kiss upon her cheek
And hold her for a while.
Because remembering her is easy,
I do it every day,
But there's an ache within my heart
That will never go away."
—Author Unknown

I miss my mom terribly, I really miss her hugs and the talks we use to have. I miss laying on her lap while she rubbed my back. There is such a huge void in my life now and I feel that I lost a big piece of my soul the day she died. A piece that I will never get back. Mom has and will miss out on so many things because of death by breast cancer treatments. I hate the very thought of cancer. It left my mom very weak and made her feel virtually powerless. It made her suffer. Then, it ravaged my mother's body and the treatments of it, finally, but ever so slowly, took her life. To me, cancer is a thief and a murderer. It will never, ever be judged and tried by a jury of its peers. It will never be given a sentence of death. It will never serve time. It is a murderer for all time, and it will continue to be so. I hate the very thought of cancer because it took my beautiful and sweet mother away from me. It committed murder without a conscience, and got away with it; and I will never forgive it for doing so.

My journey without mom has been one of turmoil and pain, but along the way I discovered that if I hugged the pain of my loss, this would be a big step toward my happiness and peace, and yours too. Although my mother's brief life's journey on Earth ended, mine did not. My new life's journey began. And as hard as it is to accept, I realize that my grief will never end. I can control it, but I will never get over feeling the loss and sadness of missing my dearly beloved mother. Over time, it has gotten better, and it will get better for you as well. There are tears that still come when I least expect it. These tears eventually turn into smiles and joyful laughter remembering all of those sweet and precious memories mom and I shared. Sometimes though, these same memories bring back all of the sadness and pain that make me miss her more and more. Please remember that although your loved one is gone, she did not leave you. She is in your heart forever. Your mother is always with you. Ask yourself what your mother would say to you about carrying on. I think my mother would say, do not be afraid to laugh, love and live your life to the fullest.

I had to learn to be honest with myself, which I found very hard to do. I had to become healthier and stronger both mentally and physically. There is a quote that always come to my mind when I am struggling and trying to figure things out. It is, "To get hat you've never had, you must do what you've never done." I live by this quote and so should you.

I am not a doctor by any means—just a daughter, published author and poet who lost her mother. I am humbled by the privilege of sharing my experience with you. From the moment my mother died, I said to myself, "How do I go on?" The answer for you and I is that you just do. You will get through it on a day-by-day basis. What choice do you have? What choice do I have? And, why do we do it? The answer is really very simple. The everlasting love that we have for our mothers.

One of the best things I ever did for my mother was to write a poem in honor of her. My first published poem is entitled: "My Mother Inside". I also honored my mother by completing and graduating with my Master of Arts degree in English, on May 17, 1997, at Southeast Missouri State University. I dropped out of graduate school to help care for my ailing mother, then two years after her death, I decided to go back and finish my college degree. She would always say to me, "In this life, you may get only one chance to do something good, so whatever you start in this life, you must finish."

Although my beautiful and sweet mother is gone, here are some other ways that I keep her memory and legacy alive and honor her:

1. Light a candle. You can do this at church and say a prayer, or like me, I sometimes light a candle at home and feel the warmth of her memory.
2. If you or somebody you know is good at quilting, make a quilt out of some of your mom's old clothes.
3. In the top of my mom's closet is a quilt she started. I have put this on my to-do list to finish.
4. Take care of your mother's grave. Every holiday and birthday, I bring flowers to my mother's grave and keep the area well-attended.
5. Cook your mom's favorite meal. Although I am not much of a cook, I can cook greens. This was one of my mom's favorite dishes. The aroma and taste brings back amazing memories of her.

6. Make a scrapbook of your mom's amazing life. I have so many pictures and personal items of my mother's. I can't wait to get started.
7. I know that we are in the tattoo era, so I am thinking about getting a tattoo of my mother's name put on the left side of my chest, close to my heart. Get a mom's tattoo for yourself!
8. Do something that your mom loved doing. Mom loved to garden, so every summer since her death I plant flowers, and rose bushes in memory of her.
9. Read your mom's favorite novel. My mom loved to read science fiction novels. Her favorite was the "The Fly". I have never read this novel, but I plan to.
10. Donate to a charity in your mother's name. I donated to The Cancer Foundation, in my mother's name.
11. Wear your mom's favorite perfume. One of my mom's favorite was Youth Dew by Estee' Lauder. I found a bottle of it in storage and I spray some on occasionally.

12. Live your life in a way that would make your mom proud. Have adventures and be happy. It is what your mom would have wanted for you. It is what I want for you.
13. Frame something that your mom has written, like a recipe.
14. Make amends with someone you have been avoiding. For me it was my mother's oncologist.
15. Sing your mother's favorite song. My mother's favorite song was "Just Coolin", by Levert.
16. Write a letter or perhaps a book about anything left unsaid. This is a helpful activity for healing.

I have learned that in grief it is important to externalize emotions. Feelings can get trapped in our bodies as our mind cycles through the same story over and over again. Writing through the grief is one way to get that repetitious story out of our bodies. For me I felt like once I had documented my story on paper, my body and mind no longer had to hold it. It helped me to feel free to move forward and find healing—I was no longer responsible for carrying my story. I went from the broken place of sadness to a life of peace and happiness, and so will you!

17. And finally, complete you mom's bucket list. My mom always wanted to travel. So now that I am retired, I plan on traveling around the world.

Doing the things that I mentioned above keeps me grounded and strong in spirit. It gives me a happy feeling inside and helps me to honor my mom and live my life to the fullest. It will do the same for you, as well!

I wrote MY JOURNEY WITHOUT MOM because I wanted to express my feelings about my mother's death in a safe and secure way. I needed to heal and writing this book was the best way for me to do that. My hope is that this book helped you through your journey in some way, answered a question or two, helped you deal with difficult feelings that you may be having, or helped you gain compassion and understanding for others going through this experience. If that hope is realized, my mom's legacy will be surely cemented in place. My mother would be delighted in knowing that she helped someone. To sum up these last twenty-three years: there has been pain, sadness, emptiness, a lot of tears, depression, laughter, smiles, and memories.

Remember, in order for you to become the strong and happy person that your mom always wanted you to be you must focus all of your energy on this one thing: forgetting the past and looking forward to what lies ahead. I had to forgive cancer for taking my mother's life and leaving me motherless. This was not an easy task. But I did it, and now I am happy and at peace. You will be also! You probably already know that God will not forgive you if you do not forgive yourself, and others. I had to forgive myself because I thought I had failed mother. I truly believed for many years that I had not done enough to prevent my mom from dying. Although I hated it, I finally realized, that it was just my mother's time to die. Forgive and you will be forgiven. When you forgive, the burden is now on the Heavenly Father, to heal all of your negative emotions, and allow peace and happiness to come onto your life.

Say to yourself every morning that today is going to be a great day. I can handle more than I think I can. Things never get better by worrying about them. There is satisfaction in knowing I did my best for my mother. There is always something to be happy about. I am going to make someone happy today. Life is great; make the most of it and simply be optimistic about the future.

My mom will forever be in my heart. Mom always gave me unconditional love and I always gave it right back. I am honored that I got to take care of my mother. I would not have had it any other way!

My mother, the bravest person I have ever known, remained strong through it all. She stayed so positive you never knew if she was just trying to keep us from feeling sad. My mom never wanted us to be angry or mad with her. She was a serious, but fun loving person. She just wanted to love and be loved, and she truly was. When I lost mom, I thought of something she would always say, "There is always some shit in the game", meaning that in this life expected the unexpected.

My mother was there when I took my first breath, and I wanted to be there for her last. This is something that I will always regret. One thing is certain though; God gave me the mother of my dreams. Mom, you will forever be my always! You are my best friend and I will always love you.

May peace and happiness be with you always!

Chapter Ten—My Love Letter To MOM

Those we love don't go away, they walk beside us every day…unseen, unheard, but always near, still loved, still missed and very dear.
—Author Unknown

My love letter to mom is about my journey without her, the love that I still have for her, and the changes that have occurred in my life since her death. As I write this letter, I keep you in mind. It is my fondest desire that you are now in a safe place where you have released the pain of losing your mother and have found the peace and happiness that you truly deserve. As you read my love letter to mom, I hope you will reflect on the everlasting love that you have for your mom and how the loss of her has finally helped you to overcome the pain, heal, and live a happier and more productive life. My Love Letter To My Mom is as follows:

Hey Mom,

How is the weather in heaven? Is it sunny and beautiful? It has been very hot here lately. I was just thinking about you and thought I'd write. Mom, I really miss you. My life is going really well and I wish you were here to be a part of it. Mother you would be pleased to hear that I have retired from teaching and I am now a published author. Seriously, Mom, I am. My book, My Journey Without Mom, is all about loving and missing you, and finding the strength to go on without you. It will be released on October 16, my birthday.

Mom, I would just like to say, "Thank you", for being my mother, loving me, and giving me the courage to pursue my dreams. And as you know, I always wanted to be a published author, and now I am. Hallelujah! You are still helping me mom. You are the inspiration that helped me write this book. Thanks to you Mom, this book will serve religious motherless daughters everywhere who have lost their mothers to cancer and are ready to go from grief-stricken to full of hope. It is full of strategies and helpful tips designed to bring comfort and understanding to those of us who are still coping with the loss of our beloved mothers.

I also write this letter to let you know that I haven't entirely accepted your death. I am still broken. My constant mourning has lessened over the years, but an incredible fear of death has taken its place. Even the mere thought of death horrifies me. My only joy is that I will be reunited with you one day. Fearing death has begun to play an increasingly important role in how I live my life, now. I think very seriously about what is important and meaningful, to me. And, with all of the pain and suffering that losing you caused, I have finally found the strength to move forward and get the peace and happiness, that I truly deserve.

Mom, please make a special effort to be with me this Tuesday, when my book is released. I would love some inside advice from you on how well it is doing. I love you Mom. Please send a kiss to dad and the rest of us. Give my love to Ella Lee, Jessie Mae, Dorothy Jean, and Ronnie Glenn. I feel better knowing they're in Heaven with you. I envy them for that. If you are not too busy cooking, please keep in touch and let me know that you received my letter—I'm not sure when it will be delivered to you.

With everlasting love always,

    Christine

My love letter to my mom is not just a letter about loving my mom who died, it is also about survival. Surviving a great loss. I survived this great loss by hugging the pain, and releasing the grief, and so will you. I live happily and peacefully now because of the life I have created. My wish is that for you, who is on a journey without mom.

I encourage you to arm yourself against pain by putting into action the strategies and tips in this book, you will add years to your life and life to your years!

Acknowledgement

I would like to begin by acknowledging and thanking my Lord and Savior Jesus Christ, from which all blessings flow. Thank you so very much Jesus for placing my feet upon this path and allowing me to become the published author I am today. Psalm119:105: Your word is a lamp to guide my feet and a light for my path. Dear Lord thank you for leading me through this journey. You guided my footsteps each day, and I did not stray from the direction you set for me, your child. Thank you Jesus! Hallelujah!

I would also like to gratefully acknowledge various people who have journeyed with me in recent weeks as I have worked on this book. First, I owe an enormous debt of gratitude to my one-hundred year old dad, Jessie Jones, for all of his love and support throughout my teaching career, and my life. Thanks dad, I love you. Secondly, I would like to thank Brady Lewis and fellow published author, Rhonda Kaalund, who have been a source of inspiration for me since I began writing my book. Rhonda introduced me to The Author's Way Program, and I have been writing forward ever since. Thank you so very much Rhonda and Brady! Thirdly, I would like to thank everyone at The Author Incubator. Without you guys, my dream to be a published author would not have been realized. May God richly bless you all.

Next, I would also like to acknowledge my third grade teacher, Mrs. Octavia Cooper and my high school English teacher, Mrs. Mary Sue McKay, who each helped me discover the love of writing. Hugs to you both. Finally, a big shout out goes to all of my English instructors at Southeast Missouri State University. My academic encounter there prepared me for becoming the published author I am today. Thank you all so very, very much!

And a final thank you to you! For believing in yourself enough to read this book. If you are reading this book, you are officially transitioning from a world of grief and pain to one of happiness and peace. What happens next —if you claw your way out of the lost and sadness and become the happy and fulfilled person your mom always wanted you to be—that's up to you. But I hope you choose happiness and peace. Remember, release the grief and find the peace, and then and only then will you have the life you have always wanted.

About The Author
Ms. Christine Jones M.A.

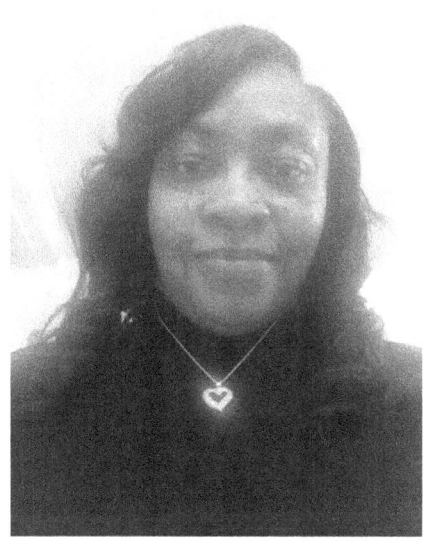

Christine Jones is a retired English teacher, published author of the book, "My Journey Without Mom" and published poet of the poem, "My Mother Inside". 'Helping young writers to write' is her motto. Christine has taught writing and worked with hundreds of students in the last 30 years. Her area of specialization is Language Acquisition and Usage. She passionately believes that writing is the pathway to the soul.

She was an item writer for DESE, (Department of Elementary and Secondary Education) for the state of Missouri, for a number of years. She was the County-Wide Spelling Bee Coordinator until her retirement. In 2000, Christine helped to write the Safe Schools Curriculum for the Hayti R-II School District. In 2005, Christine was recognized by the National Honor Roll for Outstanding American Teachers for making a positive difference in her student's lives. She served on the Professional Development Committee for the Hayti R-II School District for a number of years. Christine was also voted Who's Who Among American Women and was nominated for the Walt Disney Teacher Award. In 1983, she became vice-president of the Missouri State Teacher Association. She was also a mentor for new teachers.

In 1985, Christine received her Bachelor of Science degree in Elementary Education, and in 1997, her Masters of Arts degree in English from Southeast Missouri State University. She was on the Dean's List, with a 4.0 average.

After graduating from Southeast Missouri State University in 1985, Christine returned home to Hayti, Missouri and began her 30 year teaching career, in the Hayti R-II School District. She retired from teaching in 2017.

Christine excelled at changing her students' lives through writing. She provided a safe classroom environment and made learning fun, stimulating and engaging which was pivotal to her students' academic success. She inspired her students to work hard and pursue their dreams. She was also a trusted source of advice for students weighing important life decisions. She lives with her dad, Jessie, who is 100 years old, in the small town of Hayti, Missouri. If you blink you will miss it!

Thank You

Thank you for purchasing my book. You'll find this book to be useful in hugging the pain, releasing the grief, and finding peace and happiness. You can share this book with family, friends and coworkers. The grieving process is a challenging task for anyone to handle by themselves when it comes to the loss a loved one to cancer or death itself. Therefore, you can embrace the journey and benefit from the helpful tips in My Journey Without Mom, to overcome grief from the loss of a loved one to find happiness and peace. May GOD be with you always!

You can follow me on Facebook, Instagram, tweeter or at thechristinejones.com. When you register your email address with the www.thechristinejones.com , we will send you information about my beta groups, seminars and podcast schedules when they become available.

Notes